SUGAR IMPACT DIET JOURNAL
The Handy Companion to Track Your Progress

ISBN-13: 978-1505633313
ISBN-10: 1505633311

©2014 My Personal Journals
www.remarkableauthor.com/mpj

Free Gift for You

To get your free copy of

"How to Stay Motivated
and Lose Weight"

visit

www.staymotivatedclub.com/sugarimpact

MEASURING YOUR SUCCESS

Progress Chart

	Weight	Loss	Overall Quiz Results
Week 1			
Week 2			
Week 3			
Week 4			
Week 5			
Week 6			
Week 7			
Week 8			
Week 9			
Week 10			
Total Loss			

Body Measurements Chart

Measurement	Week 1	Week 3	Week 5	Week 7	Week 9	Inches Lost
Bust						
Chest						
Waist						
Hips						
Thigh						
Calves						
Upper arm						
Forearm						

BEFORE PICTURE

MY WEIGHT _____

WHAT I'M THINKING/HOW I FEEL: _____
_____
_____
_____
_____
_____
_____
_____

RULES TO FOLLOW

RULES TO FOLLOW

WEEKLY MEAL PLANNER
Week of _____

	BREAKFAST	LUNCH	DINNER	SNACKS
MON				
TUE				
WED				
THU				
FRI				
SAT				
SUN				

DAY 1 – Date_____

CYCLE: ☐ TAPER ☐ TRANSITION ☐ TRANSFORM

WAKE UP TIME:_____

	🕐	FOOD ITEM	TOTAL GRAMS		
			SUGAR	FRUCTOSE	CARBS
MEAL 1					
MEAL 2					
MEAL 3					

SYMPTOM IMPROVEMENTS

MY NOTES

DAY 2 – Date_____

CYCLE: ☐ TAPER ☐ TRANSITION ☐ TRANSFORM

WAKE UP TIME:_____

	🕐	FOOD ITEM	TOTAL GRAMS		
			SUGAR	FRUCTOSE	CARBS
MEAL 1					
MEAL 2					
MEAL 3					

SYMPTOM IMPROVEMENTS

MY NOTES

DAY 3 – Date_____

CYCLE: ☐ TAPER ☐ TRANSITION ☐ TRANSFORM

WAKE UP TIME:_____

	🕐	FOOD ITEM	TOTAL GRAMS		
			SUGAR	FRUCTOSE	CARBS
MEAL 1					
MEAL 2					
MEAL 3					

SYMPTOM IMPROVEMENTS

MY NOTES

DAY 4 – Date_____

CYCLE: ☐ TAPER ☐ TRANSITION ☐ TRANSFORM

WAKE UP TIME:_____

	🕐	FOOD ITEM	TOTAL GRAMS		
			SUGAR	FRUCTOSE	CARBS
MEAL 1					
MEAL 2					
MEAL 3					

SYMPTOM IMPROVEMENTS

MY NOTES

DAY 5 – Date_____

CYCLE: ☐ TAPER ☐ TRANSITION ☐ TRANSFORM

WAKE UP TIME:_____

	🕐	FOOD ITEM	TOTAL GRAMS		
			SUGAR	FRUCTOSE	CARBS
MEAL 1					
MEAL 2					
MEAL 3					

SYMPTOM IMPROVEMENTS

MY NOTES

_____   _____

_____   _____

_____   _____

DAY 6 – Date_____

CYCLE: ☐ TAPER ☐ TRANSITION ☐ TRANSFORM

WAKE UP TIME:_____

	🕐	FOOD ITEM	TOTAL GRAMS		
			SUGAR	FRUCTOSE	CARBS
MEAL 1					
MEAL 2					
MEAL 3					

SYMPTOM IMPROVEMENTS

MY NOTES

DAY 7 – Date_____

CYCLE: ☐ TAPER ☐ TRANSITION ☐ TRANSFORM

WAKE UP TIME:_____

	🕐	FOOD ITEM	TOTAL GRAMS		
			SUGAR	FRUCTOSE	CARBS
MEAL 1					
MEAL 2					
MEAL 3					

SYMPTOM IMPROVEMENTS

MY NOTES

_____   _____
_____   _____
_____   _____

WEEKLY MEAL PLANNER
Week of _____

	BREAKFAST	LUNCH	DINNER	SNACKS
MON				
TUE				
WED				
THU				
FRI				
SAT				
SUN				

DAY 8 – Date_____

CYCLE: ☐ TAPER ☐ TRANSITION ☐ TRANSFORM

WAKE UP TIME:_____

	🕒	FOOD ITEM	TOTAL GRAMS		
			SUGAR	FRUCTOSE	CARBS
MEAL 1					
MEAL 2					
MEAL 3					

SYMPTOM IMPROVEMENTS

MY NOTES

DAY 9 – Date_____

CYCLE: ☐ TAPER ☐ TRANSITION ☐ TRANSFORM

WAKE UP TIME:_____

	🕐	FOOD ITEM	TOTAL GRAMS		
			SUGAR	FRUCTOSE	CARBS
MEAL 1					
MEAL 2					
MEAL 3					

SYMPTOM IMPROVEMENTS

MY NOTES

DAY 10 – Date_____

CYCLE: ☐ TAPER ☐ TRANSITION ☐ TRANSFORM

WAKE UP TIME:_____

	🕐	FOOD ITEM	TOTAL GRAMS		
			SUGAR	FRUCTOSE	CARBS
MEAL 1					
MEAL 2					
MEAL 3					

SYMPTOM IMPROVEMENTS

MY NOTES

DAY 11 – Date_____

CYCLE: ☐ TAPER ☐ TRANSITION ☐ TRANSFORM

WAKE UP TIME:_____

	🕐	FOOD ITEM	TOTAL GRAMS		
			SUGAR	FRUCTOSE	CARBS
MEAL 1					
MEAL 2					
MEAL 3					

SYMPTOM IMPROVEMENTS

MY NOTES

DAY 12 – Date_____

CYCLE: ☐ TAPER ☐ TRANSITION ☐ TRANSFORM

WAKE UP TIME:_____

	🕐	FOOD ITEM	TOTAL GRAMS		
			SUGAR	FRUCTOSE	CARBS
MEAL 1					
MEAL 2					
MEAL 3					

SYMPTOM IMPROVEMENTS

MY NOTES

DAY 13 – Date_____

CYCLE: ☐ TAPER ☐ TRANSITION ☐ TRANSFORM

WAKE UP TIME:_____

	🕐	FOOD ITEM	TOTAL GRAMS		
			SUGAR	FRUCTOSE	CARBS
MEAL 1					
MEAL 2					
MEAL 3					

SYMPTOM IMPROVEMENTS

MY NOTES

DAY 14 – Date_____

CYCLE: ☐ TAPER ☐ TRANSITION ☐ TRANSFORM

WAKE UP TIME:_____

		FOOD ITEM	TOTAL GRAMS		
			SUGAR	FRUCTOSE	CARBS
MEAL 1					
MEAL 2					
MEAL 3					

SYMPTOM IMPROVEMENTS

MY NOTES

WEEKLY MEAL PLANNER
Week of _____

	BREAKFAST	LUNCH	DINNER	SNACKS
MON				
TUE				
WED				
THU				
FRI				
SAT				
SUN				

DAY 15 – Date_____

CYCLE: ☐ TAPER ☐ TRANSITION ☐ TRANSFORM

WAKE UP TIME:_____

	🕐	FOOD ITEM	TOTAL GRAMS		
			SUGAR	FRUCTOSE	CARBS
MEAL 1					
MEAL 2					
MEAL 3					

SYMPTOM IMPROVEMENTS

MY NOTES

DAY 16 – Date_____

CYCLE: ☐ TAPER ☐ TRANSITION ☐ TRANSFORM

WAKE UP TIME:_____

	🕐	FOOD ITEM	TOTAL GRAMS		
			SUGAR	FRUCTOSE	CARBS
MEAL 1					
MEAL 2					
MEAL 3					

SYMPTOM IMPROVEMENTS

MY NOTES

DAY 17 – Date_____

CYCLE: ☐ TAPER ☐ TRANSITION ☐ TRANSFORM

WAKE UP TIME: _____

	🕐	FOOD ITEM	TOTAL GRAMS		
			SUGAR	FRUCTOSE	CARBS
MEAL 1					
MEAL 2					
MEAL 3					

SYMPTOM IMPROVEMENTS

MY NOTES

DAY 18 – Date_____

CYCLE: ☐ TAPER ☐ TRANSITION ☐ TRANSFORM

WAKE UP TIME: _____

	🕐	FOOD ITEM	TOTAL GRAMS		
			SUGAR	FRUCTOSE	CARBS
MEAL 1					
MEAL 2					
MEAL 3					

SYMPTOM IMPROVEMENTS

MY NOTES

DAY 19 – Date_____

CYCLE: ☐ TAPER ☐ TRANSITION ☐ TRANSFORM

WAKE UP TIME: _____

	🕐	FOOD ITEM	TOTAL GRAMS		
			SUGAR	FRUCTOSE	CARBS
MEAL 1					
MEAL 2					
MEAL 3					

SYMPTOM IMPROVEMENTS

MY NOTES

DAY 20 – Date_____

CYCLE: ☐ TAPER ☐ TRANSITION ☐ TRANSFORM

WAKE UP TIME: _____

	🕐	FOOD ITEM	TOTAL GRAMS		
			SUGAR	FRUCTOSE	CARBS
MEAL 1					
MEAL 2					
MEAL 3					

SYMPTOM IMPROVEMENTS

MY NOTES

DAY 21 – Date_____

CYCLE: ☐ TAPER ☐ TRANSITION ☐ TRANSFORM

WAKE UP TIME:_____

		FOOD ITEM	TOTAL GRAMS		
			SUGAR	FRUCTOSE	CARBS
MEAL 1					
MEAL 2					
MEAL 3					

SYMPTOM IMPROVEMENTS

MY NOTES

WEEKLY MEAL PLANNER
Week of _____

	BREAKFAST	LUNCH	DINNER	SNACKS
MON				
TUE				
WED				
THU				
FRI				
SAT				
SUN				

DAY 22 – Date_____

CYCLE: ☐ TAPER ☐ TRANSITION ☐ TRANSFORM

WAKE UP TIME:_____

		FOOD ITEM	TOTAL GRAMS		
			SUGAR	FRUCTOSE	CARBS
MEAL 1					
MEAL 2					
MEAL 3					

SYMPTOM IMPROVEMENTS

MY NOTES

DAY 23 – Date_____

CYCLE: ☐ TAPER ☐ TRANSITION ☐ TRANSFORM

WAKE UP TIME: _____

	🕐	FOOD ITEM	TOTAL GRAMS		
			SUGAR	FRUCTOSE	CARBS
MEAL 1					
MEAL 2					
MEAL 3					

SYMPTOM IMPROVEMENTS

MY NOTES

DAY 24 – Date_____

CYCLE: ☐ TAPER ☐ TRANSITION ☐ TRANSFORM

WAKE UP TIME:_____

	🕐	FOOD ITEM	TOTAL GRAMS		
			SUGAR	FRUCTOSE	CARBS
MEAL 1					
MEAL 2					
MEAL 3					

SYMPTOM IMPROVEMENTS

MY NOTES

_____ _____
_____ _____
_____ _____

DAY 25 – Date_____

CYCLE: ☐ TAPER ☐ TRANSITION ☐ TRANSFORM

WAKE UP TIME:_____

	🕒	FOOD ITEM	TOTAL GRAMS		
			SUGAR	FRUCTOSE	CARBS
MEAL 1					
MEAL 2					
MEAL 3					

SYMPTOM IMPROVEMENTS

MY NOTES

DAY 26 – Date_____

CYCLE: ☐ TAPER ☐ TRANSITION ☐ TRANSFORM

WAKE UP TIME: _____

	🕐	FOOD ITEM	TOTAL GRAMS		
			SUGAR	FRUCTOSE	CARBS
MEAL 1					
MEAL 2					
MEAL 3					

SYMPTOM IMPROVEMENTS   **MY NOTES**

36

DAY 27 – Date_____

CYCLE: ☐ TAPER ☐ TRANSITION ☐ TRANSFORM

WAKE UP TIME:_____

	🕐	FOOD ITEM	TOTAL GRAMS		
			SUGAR	FRUCTOSE	CARBS
MEAL 1					
MEAL 2					
MEAL 3					

SYMPTOM IMPROVEMENTS

MY NOTES

DAY 28 – Date_____

CYCLE: ☐ TAPER ☐ TRANSITION ☐ TRANSFORM

WAKE UP TIME:_____

		FOOD ITEM	TOTAL GRAMS		
			SUGAR	FRUCTOSE	CARBS
MEAL 1					
MEAL 2					
MEAL 3					

SYMPTOM IMPROVEMENTS

MY NOTES

WEEKLY MEAL PLANNER
Week of _____

	BREAKFAST	LUNCH	DINNER	SNACKS
MON				
TUE				
WED				
THU				
FRI				
SAT				
SUN				

DAY 29 – Date_____

CYCLE: □ TAPER □ TRANSITION □ TRANSFORM

WAKE UP TIME:_____

	🕐	FOOD ITEM	TOTAL GRAMS		
			SUGAR	FRUCTOSE	CARBS
MEAL 1					
MEAL 2					
MEAL 3					

SYMPTOM IMPROVEMENTS

MY NOTES

DAY 30 – Date_____

CYCLE: ☐ TAPER ☐ TRANSITION ☐ TRANSFORM

WAKE UP TIME:_____

	🕐	FOOD ITEM	TOTAL GRAMS		
			SUGAR	FRUCTOSE	CARBS
MEAL 1					
MEAL 2					
MEAL 3					

SYMPTOM IMPROVEMENTS

MY NOTES

MIDWAY PICTURE

MY WEIGHT_____
WHAT I'M THINKING/HOW I FEEL: _____

_____
_____
_____
_____
_____
_____

DAY 31 – Date_____

CYCLE: ☐ TAPER ☐ TRANSITION ☐ TRANSFORM

WAKE UP TIME:_____

	🕐	FOOD ITEM	TOTAL GRAMS		
			SUGAR	FRUCTOSE	CARBS
MEAL 1					
MEAL 2					
MEAL 3					

SYMPTOM IMPROVEMENTS

MY NOTES

DAY 32 – Date_____

CYCLE: ☐ TAPER ☐ TRANSITION ☐ TRANSFORM

WAKE UP TIME:_____

	🕐	FOOD ITEM	TOTAL GRAMS		
			SUGAR	FRUCTOSE	CARBS
MEAL 1					
MEAL 2					
MEAL 3					

SYMPTOM IMPROVEMENTS

MY NOTES

DAY 33 – Date_____

CYCLE: ☐ TAPER ☐ TRANSITION ☐ TRANSFORM

WAKE UP TIME:_____

	🕐	FOOD ITEM	TOTAL GRAMS		
			SUGAR	FRUCTOSE	CARBS
MEAL 1					
MEAL 2					
MEAL 3					

SYMPTOM IMPROVEMENTS

MY NOTES

DAY 34 – Date_____

CYCLE: ☐ TAPER ☐ TRANSITION ☐ TRANSFORM

WAKE UP TIME:_____

	🕐	FOOD ITEM	TOTAL GRAMS		
			SUGAR	FRUCTOSE	CARBS
MEAL 1					
MEAL 2					
MEAL 3					

SYMPTOM IMPROVEMENTS

MY NOTES

DAY 35 – Date_____

CYCLE: ☐ TAPER ☐ TRANSITION ☐ TRANSFORM

WAKE UP TIME:_____

	🕐	FOOD ITEM	TOTAL GRAMS		
			SUGAR	FRUCTOSE	CARBS
MEAL 1					
MEAL 2					
MEAL 3					

SYMPTOM IMPROVEMENTS

MY NOTES

_____   _____
_____   _____
_____   _____

This page intentionally left blank

WEEKLY MEAL PLANNER
Week of _____

	BREAKFAST	LUNCH	DINNER	SNACKS
MON				
TUE				
WED				
THU				
FRI				
SAT				
SUN				

DAY 36 – Date_____

CYCLE: ☐ TAPER ☐ TRANSITION ☐ TRANSFORM

WAKE UP TIME:_____

	🕒	FOOD ITEM	TOTAL GRAMS		
			SUGAR	FRUCTOSE	CARBS
MEAL 1					
MEAL 2					
MEAL 3					

SYMPTOM IMPROVEMENTS

MY NOTES

DAY 37 – Date_____

CYCLE: ☐ TAPER ☐ TRANSITION ☐ TRANSFORM

WAKE UP TIME:_____

	🕐	FOOD ITEM	TOTAL GRAMS		
			SUGAR	FRUCTOSE	CARBS
MEAL 1					
MEAL 2					
MEAL 3					

SYMPTOM IMPROVEMENTS

MY NOTES

DAY 38 – Date_____

CYCLE: ☐ TAPER ☐ TRANSITION ☐ TRANSFORM

WAKE UP TIME:_____

	🕐	FOOD ITEM	TOTAL GRAMS		
			SUGAR	FRUCTOSE	CARBS
MEAL 1					
MEAL 2					
MEAL 3					

SYMPTOM IMPROVEMENTS

MY NOTES

DAY 39 – Date_____

CYCLE: ☐ TAPER ☐ TRANSITION ☐ TRANSFORM

WAKE UP TIME:_____

	🕐	FOOD ITEM	TOTAL GRAMS		
			SUGAR	FRUCTOSE	CARBS
MEAL 1					
MEAL 2					
MEAL 3					

SYMPTOM IMPROVEMENTS

MY NOTES

DAY 40 – Date_____

CYCLE: ☐ TAPER ☐ TRANSITION ☐ TRANSFORM

WAKE UP TIME:_____

	🕐	FOOD ITEM	TOTAL GRAMS		
			SUGAR	FRUCTOSE	CARBS
MEAL 1					
MEAL 2					
MEAL 3					

SYMPTOM IMPROVEMENTS

MY NOTES

DAY 41 – Date_____

CYCLE: ☐ TAPER ☐ TRANSITION ☐ TRANSFORM

WAKE UP TIME:_____

	🕐	FOOD ITEM	TOTAL GRAMS		
			SUGAR	FRUCTOSE	CARBS
MEAL 1					
MEAL 2					
MEAL 3					

SYMPTOM IMPROVEMENTS

MY NOTES

DAY 42 – Date_____

CYCLE: ☐ TAPER ☐ TRANSITION ☐ TRANSFORM

WAKE UP TIME:_____

	🕐	FOOD ITEM	TOTAL GRAMS		
			SUGAR	FRUCTOSE	CARBS
MEAL 1					
MEAL 2					
MEAL 3					

SYMPTOM IMPROVEMENTS

MY NOTES

WEEKLY MEAL PLANNER
Week of _____

	BREAKFAST	LUNCH	DINNER	SNACKS
MON				
TUE				
WED				
THU				
FRI				
SAT				
SUN				

DAY 43 – Date_____

CYCLE: ☐ TAPER ☐ TRANSITION ☐ TRANSFORM

WAKE UP TIME:_____

	🕐	FOOD ITEM	TOTAL GRAMS		
			SUGAR	FRUCTOSE	CARBS
MEAL 1					
MEAL 2					
MEAL 3					

SYMPTOM IMPROVEMENTS

MY NOTES

DAY 44 – Date_____

CYCLE: ☐ TAPER ☐ TRANSITION ☐ TRANSFORM

WAKE UP TIME:_____

	🕐	FOOD ITEM	TOTAL GRAMS		
			SUGAR	FRUCTOSE	CARBS
MEAL 1					
MEAL 2					
MEAL 3					

SYMPTOM IMPROVEMENTS

MY NOTES

_____ _____

_____ _____

_____ _____

DAY 45 – Date_____

CYCLE: ☐ TAPER ☐ TRANSITION ☐ TRANSFORM

WAKE UP TIME:_____

	🕐	FOOD ITEM	TOTAL GRAMS		
			SUGAR	FRUCTOSE	CARBS
MEAL 1					
MEAL 2					
MEAL 3					

SYMPTOM IMPROVEMENTS

MY NOTES

DAY 46 – Date_____

CYCLE: ☐ TAPER ☐ TRANSITION ☐ TRANSFORM

WAKE UP TIME:_____

	🕐	FOOD ITEM	TOTAL GRAMS		
			SUGAR	FRUCTOSE	CARBS
MEAL 1					
MEAL 2					
MEAL 3					

SYMPTOM IMPROVEMENTS

MY NOTES

DAY 47 – Date_____

CYCLE: ☐ TAPER ☐ TRANSITION ☐ TRANSFORM

WAKE UP TIME:_____

	🕐	FOOD ITEM	TOTAL GRAMS		
			SUGAR	FRUCTOSE	CARBS
MEAL 1					
MEAL 2					
MEAL 3					

SYMPTOM IMPROVEMENTS

MY NOTES

DAY 48 – Date_____

CYCLE: ☐ TAPER ☐ TRANSITION ☐ TRANSFORM

WAKE UP TIME:_____

	🕐	FOOD ITEM	TOTAL GRAMS		
			SUGAR	FRUCTOSE	CARBS
MEAL 1					
MEAL 2					
MEAL 3					

SYMPTOM IMPROVEMENTS

MY NOTES

_____   _____

_____   _____

_____   _____

DAY 49 – Date_____

CYCLE: ☐ TAPER ☐ TRANSITION ☐ TRANSFORM

WAKE UP TIME: _____

	🕐	FOOD ITEM	TOTAL GRAMS		
			SUGAR	FRUCTOSE	CARBS
MEAL 1					
MEAL 2					
MEAL 3					

SYMPTOM IMPROVEMENTS

MY NOTES

WEEKLY MEAL PLANNER
Week of _____

	BREAKFAST	LUNCH	DINNER	SNACKS
MON				
TUE				
WED				
THU				
FRI				
SAT				
SUN				

DAY 50 – Date_____

CYCLE: ☐ TAPER ☐ TRANSITION ☐ TRANSFORM

WAKE UP TIME:_____

	🕐	FOOD ITEM	TOTAL GRAMS		
			SUGAR	FRUCTOSE	CARBS
MEAL 1					
MEAL 2					
MEAL 3					

SYMPTOM IMPROVEMENTS

MY NOTES

DAY 51 – Date_____

CYCLE: ☐ TAPER ☐ TRANSITION ☐ TRANSFORM

WAKE UP TIME:_____

	🕐	FOOD ITEM	TOTAL GRAMS		
			SUGAR	FRUCTOSE	CARBS
MEAL 1					
MEAL 2					
MEAL 3					

SYMPTOM IMPROVEMENTS

MY NOTES

DAY 52 – Date_____

CYCLE: ☐ TAPER ☐ TRANSITION ☐ TRANSFORM

WAKE UP TIME:_____

	🕐	FOOD ITEM	TOTAL GRAMS		
			SUGAR	FRUCTOSE	CARBS
MEAL 1					
MEAL 2					
MEAL 3					

SYMPTOM IMPROVEMENTS

MY NOTES

DAY 53 – Date_____

CYCLE: ☐ TAPER ☐ TRANSITION ☐ TRANSFORM

WAKE UP TIME: _____

	🕐	FOOD ITEM	TOTAL GRAMS		
			SUGAR	FRUCTOSE	CARBS
MEAL 1					
MEAL 2					
MEAL 3					

SYMPTOM IMPROVEMENTS

MY NOTES

DAY 54 – Date_____

CYCLE: ☐ TAPER ☐ TRANSITION ☐ TRANSFORM

WAKE UP TIME:_____

		FOOD ITEM	TOTAL GRAMS		
			SUGAR	FRUCTOSE	CARBS
MEAL 1					
MEAL 2					
MEAL 3					

SYMPTOM IMPROVEMENTS

MY NOTES

DAY 55 – Date_____

CYCLE: ☐ TAPER ☐ TRANSITION ☐ TRANSFORM

WAKE UP TIME:_____

	🕐	FOOD ITEM	TOTAL GRAMS		
			SUGAR	FRUCTOSE	CARBS
MEAL 1					
MEAL 2					
MEAL 3					

SYMPTOM IMPROVEMENTS

MY NOTES

_____ _____

_____ _____

_____ _____

DAY 56 – Date_____

CYCLE: ☐ TAPER ☐ TRANSITION ☐ TRANSFORM

WAKE UP TIME:_____

	🕐	FOOD ITEM	TOTAL GRAMS		
			SUGAR	FRUCTOSE	CARBS
MEAL 1					
MEAL 2					
MEAL 3					

SYMPTOM IMPROVEMENTS

MY NOTES

WEEKLY MEAL PLANNER
Week of _____

	BREAKFAST	LUNCH	DINNER	SNACKS
MON				
TUE				
WED				
THU				
FRI				
SAT				
SUN				

DAY 57 – Date_____

CYCLE: ☐ TAPER ☐ TRANSITION ☐ TRANSFORM

WAKE UP TIME:_____

	🕐	FOOD ITEM	TOTAL GRAMS		
			SUGAR	FRUCTOSE	CARBS
MEAL 1					
MEAL 2					
MEAL 3					

SYMPTOM IMPROVEMENTS

MY NOTES

DAY 58 – Date_____

CYCLE: ☐ TAPER ☐ TRANSITION ☐ TRANSFORM

WAKE UP TIME:_____

		FOOD ITEM	TOTAL GRAMS		
			SUGAR	FRUCTOSE	CARBS
MEAL 1					
MEAL 2					
MEAL 3					

SYMPTOM IMPROVEMENTS

MY NOTES

DAY 59 – Date_____

CYCLE: ☐ TAPER ☐ TRANSITION ☐ TRANSFORM

WAKE UP TIME:_____

	🕒	FOOD ITEM	TOTAL GRAMS		
			SUGAR	FRUCTOSE	CARBS
MEAL 1					
MEAL 2					
MEAL 3					

SYMPTOM IMPROVEMENTS

MY NOTES

DAY 60 – Date_____

CYCLE: ☐ TAPER ☐ TRANSITION ☐ TRANSFORM

WAKE UP TIME:_____

	🕐	FOOD ITEM	TOTAL GRAMS		
			SUGAR	FRUCTOSE	CARBS
MEAL 1					
MEAL 2					
MEAL 3					

SYMPTOM IMPROVEMENTS

MY NOTES

AFTER PICTURE

MY WEIGHT_____

WHAT I'M THINKING/HOW I FEEL: _____
_____
_____
_____
_____
_____
_____

FAVORITE RECIPES

Recipe Name: _____
*Serves:*_____

Oven Temp_____Prep Time_____Cook Time _____

Ingredients:

_____   _____

_____   _____

_____   _____

_____   _____

Preparation Directions:

_____
_____
_____
_____
_____

Cooking Directions:

_____
_____
_____
_____
_____

Notes:

_____
_____
_____
_____
_____

FAVORITE RECIPES

Recipe Name: _____
*Serves:*_____

Oven Temp_____ Prep Time_____ Cook Time _____

Ingredients:

Preparation Directions:

Cooking Directions:

Notes:

FAVORITE RECIPES

Recipe Name: _____
*Serves:*_____

Oven Temp_____Prep Time_____Cook Time _____

Ingredients:
_____   _____
_____   _____
_____   _____
_____   _____

Preparation Directions:
_____
_____
_____
_____
_____

Cooking Directions:
_____
_____
_____
_____
_____

Notes:
_____
_____
_____
_____
_____

FAVORITE RECIPES

Recipe Name: _____
*Serves:*_____

Oven Temp_____Prep Time_____Cook Time _____

Ingredients:
_____   _____

_____   _____

_____   _____

_____   _____

Preparation Directions:
_____
_____
_____
_____
_____

Cooking Directions:
_____
_____
_____
_____
_____

Notes:
_____
_____
_____
_____
_____

FAVORITE RECIPES

Recipe Name: _____
*Serves:*_____

Oven Temp_____Prep Time_____Cook Time _____

Ingredients:
_____   _____

_____   _____

_____   _____

_____   _____

Preparation Directions:
_____
_____
_____
_____
_____

Cooking Directions:
_____
_____
_____
_____

Notes:
_____
_____
_____
_____
_____

FAVORITE RECIPES

Recipe Name: _____
*Serves:*_____

Oven Temp_____Prep Time_____Cook Time _____

Ingredients:
_____   _____

_____   _____

_____   _____

_____   _____

Preparation Directions:
_____
_____
_____
_____
_____

Cooking Directions:
_____
_____
_____
_____
_____

Notes:
_____
_____
_____
_____
_____

FAVORITE RECIPES

Recipe Name: _____
*Serves:*_____

Oven Temp_____Prep Time_____Cook Time _____

Ingredients:
_____   _____
_____   _____
_____   _____
_____   _____

Preparation Directions:
_____
_____
_____
_____
_____

Cooking Directions:
_____
_____
_____
_____
_____

Notes:
_____
_____
_____
_____
_____

FAVORITE RECIPES

Recipe Name: _____
*Serves:*_____

Oven Temp_____ Prep Time_____ Cook Time _____

Ingredients:
_____   _____

_____   _____

_____   _____

_____   _____

Preparation Directions:
_____
_____
_____
_____
_____

Cooking Directions:
_____
_____
_____
_____
_____

Notes:
_____
_____
_____
_____
_____

NOTES

NOTES

NOTES

NOTES

SHOPPING LIST

SHOPPING LIST

SHOPPING LIST